WALKING
MY ASS OFF

T.S. Koelling

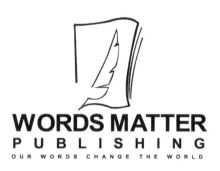

WORDS MATTER
P U B L I S H I N G
OUR WORDS CHANGE THE WORLD

© 2022 by T.S. Koelling. All rights reserved.
Words Matter Publishing
P.O. Box 531
Salem, Il 62881
www.wordsmatterpublishing.com

ISBN: 978-1-953912-62-6

Library of Congress Catalog Card Number: 2022935054

TABLE OF CONTENT

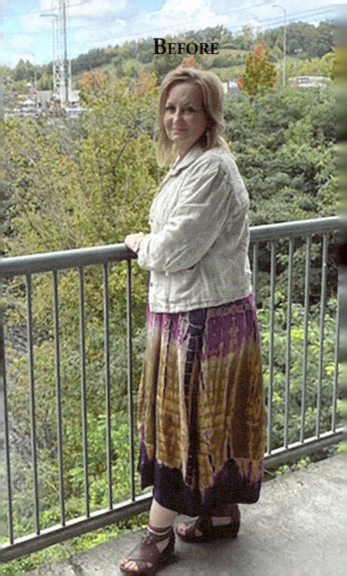

BEFORE

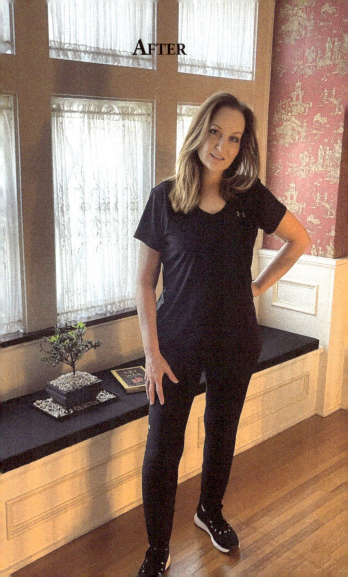

AFTER

FOREWORD

As a youth I was skin and bones ate what I wanted and didn't gain a pound. Up until my mid-30's I was 5'3" and 100 lbs fully-dressed soaking wet. By the end of my 30's I noticed a change. I was beginning to pick up weight and instead of changing my eating and exercise habits at that time I accepted the added ten pounds with a smirk when I looked in the mirror feeling I didn't have a thing to worry about. By the end of my 40's I wasn't smirking anymore because I seldom looked in a mirror that showed more than my head when I was applying makeup and doing my hair because

I didn't want to even glance at the extra 15 lbs I had picked up over the last decade. As the 50's rolled in so did an added 40 lbs and soon I was having a hard time walking up stairs and keeping up with my dog. At 165 lbs I knew I needed to do something different because I was seriously overweight for my height, so I began to consider my options.

Gym Wasn't a Win

My lifestyle didn't lend itself to workout sessions in a gym. I couldn't afford a personal trainer and didn't have a clue how to use most of the equipment, so going to the gym did not ever enter my thoughts again.

A Diet Wasn't Right

I tried a few plans and programs spent quite a bit of money and lost a few pounds that quickly reappeared the minute I ate anything that wasn't on the menu of these programs, and I hated the cardboard flavorless food.

Water Wasn't Working
Drinking 2 gallons of water each day made me feel bloated and sluggish.

Walking
I knew I needed to get moving and I had heard about walking to lose weight, so I downloaded an app on my phone called Steps App. For the next few weeks, I just let the app count my steps daily and I paid little attention to it. And then…the unthinkable happened that launched me into a lifestyle change and soon I was down 25 lbs. I was happier and looked better than I had in two decades. I had found my solution and I was dropping the pounds while eating whatever I wanted whenever I wanted it. And you can too!

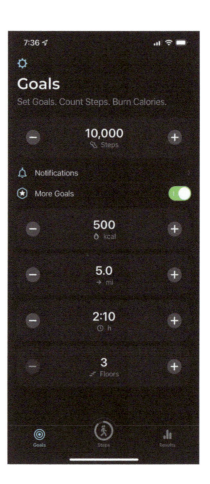

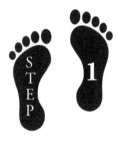

TAKING THE FIRST STEP

Opening the Steps App one day as I waited at the dentist office, I decided to see what my normal daily step count was. I had averaged 3500 steps a day, I was burning a little over 100 calories and walking a mile and a half. Not a bad start. I certainly had something that I could build on. I decided to keep it simple and doable and set my goal on 4500 steps. I also noticed the goal setting option for floors (walking up and down stairs) and since the house I was living in had a basement I added 2 floors to my daily goal plan. Just setting a reachable goal was powerful, I felt more in control of my health than I had in 30 years. I was excited to begin and wanted the dentist to hurry up!

As I left the dentist office, I took the first step to getting my weight under control. I chuckled as I realized now the hardest part would be to keep my phone on me so that my steps were accurately recorded. Easy breezy! I then decided that I would not change my eating habits yet. I wanted to begin slow and set only the goals that I knew I could reach on a consistent basis. Mentally I made a note to add a change of diet a few months down the road after I had mastered the walking part of my new lifestyle. I didn't know at that time that I would never need to change the foods that I ate because I would soon be burning more calories than I took in daily which is all I needed to do to watch the pounds come off and my body become more toned than it had been in years.

At the end of the first week, I had easily mastered the 4500 steps a day goal and immediately bumped it up to 5500. I gradually began to do more things while walking. I walked while talking to clients on the phone, I walked while watching TV, I even learned to answer emails while walking.

Your Turn to Take the First Step

1. Download the Steps App and ignore it for a week to determine what your normal daily step count is.

2. Add 1,000 steps to your average daily step count in the goal selection of the app.

3. Begin walking while talking on the phone, posting on social media etc.

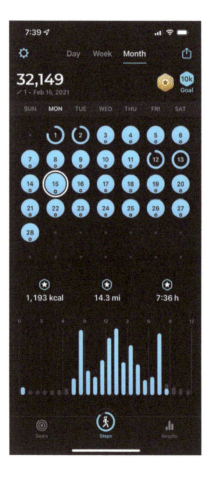

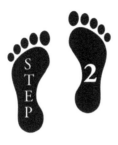

BUILDING A ROUTINE

I had just mastered 7,000 steps a day when my mother died, and my world came crumbling down. Grief overtook me and to deal with the pain I walked! For hours each day I paced the small home I was living in. One day I walked 32,149 steps, for a total of 14.3 miles and I burned 1,193 kcal. Over a period of 3 months, I had walked 1,112,880 steps, or 490 miles and burned 40,900 kcal. While dealing with my grief I had discovered several things:

1. My daily walking goal of 7,000 steps was ridiculously low.

2. Walking was a mind game. If I had set out to walk 30,000 steps a day, I would have never been able to do it. My mind would have worked against me the entire time. However, while I was walking 30,000 steps a day focusing on my mother and my life without her I wasn't tired, my legs and knees didn't hurt, and I was never out of breath.

3. I had lost 12 lbs eating junk food because I hadn't felt like cooking.

As I began to cope with the loss of my mother, I began to establish a normal walking routine consisting of 10,000 steps a day. I had read that you needed to walk 10,000 steps a day for consistent weight loss. Since I was now used to at least twice this number of steps I set the goal on my Steps App at 12,000 steps and kept it there for many months finally dialing it down to the magic number of 10,000 steps. I was now down 20 lbs.

Your Turn to Build Your Routine

1. Gradually build your steps to a daily count of 10,000. This may take several months or more but as long as you are increasing your step count 500 additional steps each week you will eventually reach the 10,000 steps a day goal.

2. Maintain your goal each day but don't get discouraged if life gets in the way and you fall short of your 10,000 steps on some days. We all have those days, what is important is that you have more

days each month of reaching your goal than days of not reaching your goal.

3. Don't let your mind get in the way just walk. Walk while reading a book (but watch where you are going). Walk while texting, watching TV, talking on the phone, and even eating. Just walk and look at your step counter a couple of times throughout the day. Don't get hung up on the number of steps you still have to go just find ways to walk while doing other things. This helps your mind to concentrate on the task you are doing and not the number of steps you still need to reach your goal for the day.

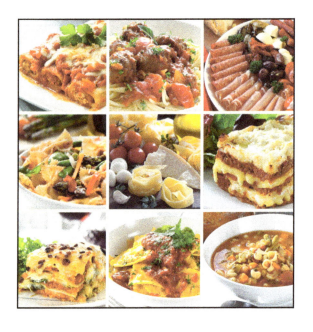

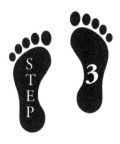

S
T
E
P

3

CREATING A CALORIC DEFICIT

Losing weight is simply a matter of burning more calories than you eat. This is called a caloric deficit. Every person is different and that is why diet and exercise programs don't work for everyone. There is no one size fits all program for losing weight except **creating a caloric deficit** which is self-explanatory when you burn more than you take in you will be burning stored fat.

As you begin to walk be mindful of what you are eating. Glance at the calories on packaging and at restaurants. I was mindful of my caloric intake, but I never wrote down the foods or calories I ate, and I certainly never pulled out the calculator. At the end of each day, I knew approximately how many calories I had taken in, and I checked to see how many calories I had burned by walking. When I mentally added in the other activities of the day that burned calories, I knew whether I had reached my goal of creating a caloric deficit for the day. The scales also knew and when my morning weigh in revealed that half pound loss the scales became my friend that rewarded me.

The best part about using a caloric deficit to lose weight is you can have that piece of Birthday cake at the office party without feeling guilty by simply walking a few more steps that day. No food is off limits! No amount of food is off limits! Just walk a little extra to compensate for the splurge and all is well.

Your Turn to create a Caloric Deficit

1. Mentally record the number of calories you are taking in each day. If you want to be more precise record your intake, but this certainly isn't required for this program to work.

2. Research the number of calories you are burning while doing your daily routine. Add this to your mental list. If you have doubts just Google it. You can find the caloric burn for most any activity online.

3. Now you will be able to determine the number of calories you need to burn from walking to reach your caloric deficit or the day. When you master this step, you are well on your way to walking your ass off!!!

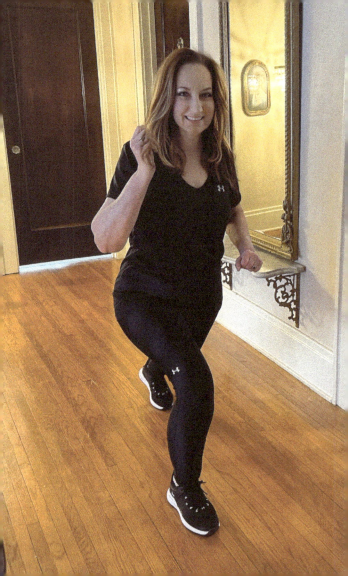

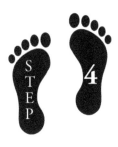

VARIATIONS

I once thought you had to really *workout* to lose inches…but you don't! As I walked the inches melted away. I did however add a few variations to my walking pattern which helped to tone my legs, hips and butt.

1. I walked backwards for 1,000 steps a day.

2. I walked in circles to the right and to the left.

3. I walked in squats (knees bent) for at least 1,000 steps a day.

4. I walked up and down stairs four to ten times a day.

By walking backwards and in circles I was able to watch movies, and TV while walking. I was also toning up muscles and skin from the loss of several inches.

Your Turn to Use Variations

1. Try some of the above variations to see what you enjoy and what works for you.

2. Come up with your own variations and have fun with it. Be creative. The goal of the variations is to add a little more to your walking routine that helps tone

your body and keeps you engaged as you walk.

3. Pick up the pace. Any speed is great but of course increasing your pace is better, but don't walk so fast that you burn out or are too tired to complete your daily step goal.

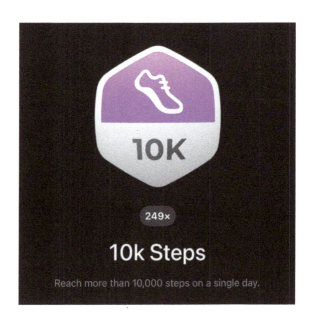

249x

10k Steps

Reach more than 10,000 steps on a single day.

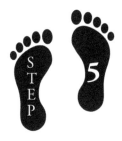

A LIFELONG HABIT

Walking became a great source of comfort to me as I was healing after losing mom. I now walk to alleviate stress and find that I'm able to walk my way through most any problem. It is an added bonus that I am able to maintain my weight loss by simply doing something that I have come to love…walking.

I think it is also important for you to know that I walk indoors unless the weather is right and I'm taking one of the dogs out. Walking is an activity you can do right in the comfort of your home even in bad weather. This is now a lifelong habit for me, and I hope it will become one for you as well. Not only will you lose the weight and inches, but your overall mental state will improve, and you'll feel better about your life than you have in years.

Because I had moved in with mom to take care of her when she reached 94, after she passed at age 98, I had to move, and I bought a home with over 8,000 square feet and eight staircases. Why would a single woman need so much space? Because walking had become a lifelong habit for me, and I had learned to thrive as I walked my ass off!

Your Turn to Make a Lifelong Habit as You Walk You Ass Off!

THE SIMPLE SOLUTION SERIES

Life is hard enough, and problems are big enough.

Solutions don't have to be complicated or costly they just need to be effective.

This series is all about offering you a simple solution to your problems in just a few steps.

In this series, I am going to **KEEP IT SIMPLE!**

Milton Keynes UK
Ingram Content Group UK Ltd.
UKHW021102201124
2888UKWH00017B/104

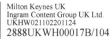

9 781953 912626